Preface

This manual provides information beyond that contained in the video it accompanies, *Understanding the Defiant Child*. That videotape is one of a two-volume set, the other being *Managing the Defiant Child* (Barkley, 1997a). This manual is intended to provide an overview of defiance in children that fills in details that could not be covered at all or in as much detail in the tape. For in-depth coverage of defiance in children, please see my clinical manual, *Defiant Children* (2nd ed.): *A Clinician's Manual for Assessment and Parent Training* (Barkley, 1997b, 1997c).

The videotape associated with this manual is designed to provide a stimulating and informative review of our current knowledge about defiance in children, a common behavior pattern that research suggests may be increasing in prevalence and that is a known precursor to more serious clinical disorders, such as oppositional defiant disorder (ODD) and conduct disorder (CD). The videotape can be used for a number of purposes:

1. To obtain further information about defiance in children.
2. To accompany a presentation to parents about this behavior pattern as part of group or individual parent

training in child behavior management methods, such as those set forth in my clinical manual, *Defiant Children*.
3. In conjunction with in-service training of educators or other professionals on defiant behavior and ODD and its management.
4. To educate parents, relatives, or teachers about defiance or ODD in children as part of clinical feedback conferences following the evaluation of a child who has defiance or ODD.
5. As part of high school, undergraduate, or graduate classes on abnormal psychology or abnormal child psychology when covering the topic of ODD or defiant behavior.
6. In conjunction with medical school or residency training in child psychiatry, pediatrics, child neurology, or family medicine, or internship/fellowship training in child clinical psychology when reviewing common childhood behavioral disorders, in particular, ODD.

As with my four videotapes on attention-deficit/hyperactivity disorder (ADHD; Barkley, 1993a, 1993b, 1994a, 1994b), I have tried to make sure that the content of this videotape is as current as possible and that it reflects the general consensus of professional and scientific opinion about the management of defiance and ODD.

This videotape is the culmination of a collaborative effort of myself, Kevin Dawkins, the producer, and the staff of The Guilford Press, in particular, Sharon Panulla, Seymour Weingarten, and Robert Matloff. I am indebted to them all, particularly Kevin and Sharon, for their splendid and creative contributions to this endeavor; Kevin's exceptional editing prowess brought the subject matter to life through the lives of families who have children with significant defiant behavior. And let me once again express my never-ending thanks to Seymour and Robert for their financial support of this project, ideas for its structure, and publication of the videotapes. The impact their publication activities have on the mental health profession and those who seek its help is enormous and probably beyond what they imagine it to be.

Understanding the Defiant Child

Program Manual

RUSSELL A. BARKLEY, PhD

THE GUILFORD PRESS
New York London

*To Constance Hanf, PhD,
Professor Emeritus
of the
Oregon Health Sciences University,
for teaching me to pay attention
to defiance and its children*

©1997 The Guilford Press
A Division of Guilford Publications, Inc.
72 Spring Street, New York, NY 10012

All rights reserved

No part of this book may be reproduced, stored in a retrieval system, or transmitted, in any form or by any means, electronic, mechanical, photocopying, microfilming, recording, or otherwise, without written permission from the Publisher.

Understanding the Defiant Child. A Program Manual.

This manual accompanies the videotape *Understanding the Defiant Child*, ©1997 by The Guilford Press.

ISBN 1-57230-166-X

Even greater appreciation must be expressed to the families and children who share their stories, successes, and failures, as well as messages of hope, on the videotapes. Without their courage to do so, the project would not have been possible. All of us who contributed to the creation of the videotapes on the defiant child owe these families a great deal of gratitude for their participation in this project.

I also appreciate the assistance of my colleagues and students who agreed to appear on the videotapes. Thanks go specifically to Gwenyth Edwards, PhD, Chief of the ADHD Clinic at the University of Massachusetts Medical Center, for sharing her wisdom about defiant children and the training of parents in effective child management methods. And I greatly appreciate the assistance of Jodi Dooling-Litfin, PhD, and William Hathaway, PhD, for their assistance in conducting the group parent training program that appears in segments of these videotapes. Last, and once more, I express my continual gratitude to my wife, Pat, and sons, Ken and Steve, for their support of me and this project.

Contents

Degrees of Noncompliance/Defiance	1
How Prevalent is Defiant Behavior or ODD?	4
Why Be Concerned About Defiant Behavior in Children	4
Important Aspects of the Interactions of Defiant Children with Their Parents	10
What Causes Defiance in Children?	16
Summary	19
Appendix	21
Suggested Readings	27
Parent Training	28

What is defiant behavior? It is generally taken to mean one of two things. One is noncompliance, or passive avoidance of following parental commands and previously stated household rules. The child simply does not perform as instructed or ignores well-established rules, sometimes without direct confrontation with the rule-giver. The second meaning of defiant behavior is overtly hostile and confrontational behavior of a child toward a parent or other authority figure. Such behavior includes displays of active verbal or physical resistance to complying with parental directives, as in the case of verbal refusal, temper outbursts, and even physical aggression against a parent when the parent attempts to impose on the child compliance with a parental directive. Examples of noncompliant and defiant behaviors are shown in Table 1. Many of the behaviors in Table 1 are in fact direct efforts of the child to escape or avoid carrying out a command. Hence, all may be treated by a single program that addresses noncompliance.

Degrees of Noncompliance/Defiance

There exist degrees of noncompliant behavior the terms for which are not always agreed on by professionals. Whereas professionals have agreed on carving mental retardation into the degrees of slow, borderline, mild, moderate, and severe or profound, no such labeling consensus exists for degrees of

TABLE 1. Types of Noncompliant Behaviors Common in Children Referred for Behavior Disorders

Yells	Steals	Physically resists
Whines	Lies	Destroys property
Complains	Argues	Physically fights with others
Defies	Humiliates/Annoys	Fails to complete school homework
Screams	Teases	Disrupts others' activities
Tantrums	Ignores requests	Ignores self-care tasks
Throws objects	Runs off	
Talks back	Cries	
Swears	Fails to complete routine chores	

Note. From Barkley (1997, p. 18). Copyright 1997 by The Guilford Press. Reprinted by permission.

noncompliant or defiant behavior (though adapting the mental retardation categories might be appropriate). Children whose defiant behavior is above average but below the 84th percentile on a standardized behavior rating scale may be considered normal even though they may be stubborn, strong-willed, opinionated, and even difficult to manage at times. Children placing above the 84th percentile but below the 93rd percentile could be described as being "noncompliant" or "defiant" or as having borderline ODD, provided they do not meet the full clinical diagnostic criteria for that disorder in the most recent *Diagnostic and Statistical Manual for Mental Disorders* (DSM-IV; American Psychiatric Association, 1994). Children who place above the 93rd percentile or who meet full clinical criteria for ODD could be said to have the disorder. The degree could be described as mild, moderate, or severe, depending on the severity of the rating, or the number of ODD symptoms a child possesses above the minimal number required to meet the diagnostic threshold. Parents of children in any of these categories except the normal one might benefit from a parent training program, such as that described in the other videotape in this series, *Managing Defiant Children*, or in my clinical manual, *Defiant Children*.

TABLE 2. Diagnostic Criteria for Oppositional Defiant Disorder

A. A pattern of negativistic, hostile, and defiant behavior lasting at least 6 months, during which four (or more) of the following are present:
   (1) often loses temper
   (2) often argues with adults
   (3) often actively defies or refuses to comply with adults' requests or rules
   (4) often deliberately annoys people
   (5) often blames others for his or her mistakes or misbehavior
   (6) is often touchy or easily annoyed by others
   (7) is often angry and resentful
   (8) is often spiteful or vindictive

Note: Consider a criterion met only if the behavior occurs more frequently than is typically observed in individuals of comparable age and developmental level.

B. The disturbance in behavior causes clinically significant impairment in social, academic, or occupational functioning.
C. The behaviors do not occur exclusively during the course of a Psychotic or Mood Disorder.
D. Criteria are not met for Conduct Disorder, and, if the individual is age 18 years or older, criteria are not met for Antisocial Personality Disorder.

Note. From American Psychiatric Association (1994, pp. 93–94). Copyright 1994 by the American Psychiatric Association. Reprinted by permission.

The current clinical diagnostic criteria for ODD, as set forth in DSM-IV, are listed in Table 2. The majority of children with ODD have attention-deficit/ hyperactivity disorder (ADHD) as a coexisting condition, so the reader may wish to become familiar with those DSM-IV diagnostic criteria.

Childhood defiance and ODD are strongly associated with a greater risk for eventual childhood conduct disorder (CD). While approximately 20 to 25 percent of children with ODD may no longer have the disorder three years later, up to 52 percent persist in having ODD. Of those who persist with ODD, nearly half (25 percent of the initial total of ODD children) progress into childhood CD and its associated patterns of delinquent, antisocial behavior and the violation of the rights of others within a 3-year follow-up period. The age of onset of early CD symptoms has been shown repeatedly to be a particularly important predictor of the progression into delinquency and the severity and persistence of such delinquency; the onset of initial symptoms before age 12 years is a particularly salient threshold in making such predictions.

How Prevalent Is Defiant Behavior or ODD?

As the foregoing discussion implies, the frequency with which children manifest clinically significant and impairing levels of defiant and noncompliant behavior is greatly determined by the definition used for such disorders when surveying childhood populations. DSM-IV cites a prevalence ranging between 2 and 16 percent for ODD. Using parent reports of child behavior problems in a large sample (1,096) of military dependents 6 to 17 years old, one study reported a prevalence of 4.9 percent for ODD. In contrast, using teacher ratings has shown a prevalence of 3.2 percent. Given the limited contexts in which teachers observe child behavior (school buildings and grounds) and that oppositional and antisocial behavior is more likely to occur at home and in the community, such prevalence rates are probably underestimates of these disorders in the population. Most studies show a sharp decline in the prevalence of ODD from childhood to adolescence, which may attest to the facts that some ODD children are maturing out of their disorder and others are progressing from ODD into CD. The sex ratios in many studies are approximately 2:1 to 3:1 (males to females) for both ODD and CD. Obviously, less clinically serious degrees of defiant behavior could be expected to occur with even greater frequency than these figures suggest.

Why Be Concerned About Defiant Behavior in Children?

Although some noncompliance and defiance in children is normal, particularly in toddlers and young preschool children, the occurence of such behavior more frequently or more severely than normal is a significant risk factor for a number of serious negative outcomes. Parents, educators, and clinical professionals should be concerned about frequent or severe instances of defiance and its underlying family processes for a number of well-established reasons.

High Proportion of Clinic Referrals

Over half of all referrals to child mental health clinics are for oppositional or aggressive behavior. A major concern of the parent or teacher referring a defiant child is the child's inability to comply with directions, commands, rules, or codes of social conduct appropriate to the child's age group. Parents complain that the child fails to listen, throws temper tantrums, is aggressive or destructive, is verbally resistant to authority, fails to do homework, does not adequately perform chores, cannot play appropriately with neighborhood children, lies or steals frequently, or shows other forms of inappropriate behavior. All these behaviors are violations of commands, directions, or rules that were either previously stated to the child or stated in the particular situation. Hence, defiance, broadly defined, encompasses the majority of acting out, externalizing, or conduct problems that lead to clinical referrals for mental health services.

High Levels of Family Conflict

Noncompliance underlies the majority of negative interactions between family members and the referred child. Disruptive or aggressive behavior by children occurs neither continuously nor randomly throughout the day but instead appears in "bursts" or "chunks" of high-rate, often intense oppositional or coercive behavior that punctuate otherwise normal behavior. Research suggests that one of the most common precipitants of child noncompliance or defiance is parental or teacher commands or requests.

Negative encounters between adult and child seem to take the form shown schematically in Figure 1 in many, though not all, instances. The sequence is initiated by a parent's command to have the child engage in a task that the child typically does not consider enjoyable or reinforcing, such as picking up toys, cleaning up his or her room, or doing school homework. On rare occasions, the behavior-disordered child obeys the first request.

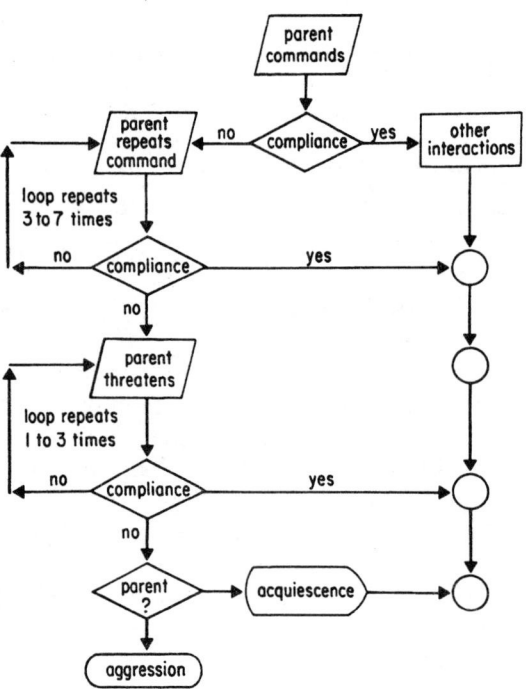

FIGURE 1. Possible sequencing of interactions between parents and defiant children during a command–compliance encounter. From Barkley (1997, p. 28). Copyright 1997 by The Guilford Press. Reprinted by permission.

Compliance usually occurs when the command involves the child in a very brief amount of effort or work (e.g., "Please hand me a Kleenex") or in an activity that is pleasurable to the child or that promises immediate reinforcement for compliance (i.e., "Get in the car so we can go get some ice cream"). As shown at the right of Figure 1, the child complies with the request and the family proceeds to other interactions.

What is significant here is that rarely does the parent socially reinforce immediate compliance, for example, by acknowledging appreciation for the compliance. When compliance goes unnoted by parents, it frequently declines in occurrence

Understanding the Defiant Child

over time and may eventually occur only when the activity requested of the child is highly intrinsically rewarding and the reward is immediately available. In such cases, the child obeys not because of having been reinforced by the parent for doing so but because the activity is reinforcing.

Yet, usually in only very few instances do defiant children comply with any first commands or requests of parents. More often, the pattern of events is that seen at the left side of Figure 1. The child fails to comply with the initial command, and the parent repeats the command to the child. The child does not comply with the second command, and the parent repeats the command as many as 5 to 15 times (or more!) in various forms—without the child complying. At some point, parental frustration rises and the emotional intensity of the interaction heightens. The parent then warns or threatens the child that if the child does not comply, something unpleasant or punitive will follow. Yet the child usually fails to comply even when threatened in part, often, because the parent repeats the threat instead of enforcing it. Over time, both parent and child escalate their level of emotional behavior toward the other, raising their voices in volume and intensity and displaying anger, defiance, or destructiveness. The interaction sequence ends in one of several ways. Less frequently, the parent disciplines the child, perhaps by sending the child to his or her room, removing a privilege, or even hitting the child. Discipline often fails because it is inconsistently applied and delayed hopelessly beyond the point where compliance was initially requested. More often, the parent gives up, and the child leaves the command uncompleted or only partially completed. Even if the child eventually does the task, however, the child has succeeded in at least delaying its completion.

Eventual child compliance presents an enigma to parents and professionals alike. Parents may believe that they have actually "won," or at least succeeded in getting the child to listen, yet they are surprised to find that the child again attempts to avoid or defy the same command when it is issued again later. Parents may ask the therapist why the child continues to misbehave or defy them when he ultimately can be forced to perform the task. The key to understanding this situation is to look at it from a child's point of view rather than an adult's.

Adults tend to look at the situation in its entirety and are able to see that ultimately they can make the child perform the command. Most children are not aware of the entire interaction sequence but simply view it as a moment-to-moment interaction with their parents in which their immediate goal is to escape or avoid doing the requested task, even if only temporarily; every minute the child can procrastinate is an additional minute the child can continue to do what he or she was doing prior to the imposition of the command—usually an activity more reinforcing to the child than the one the parents wish him or her to do. It is also an additional minute of avoiding the often unpleasant task requested by the parent; avoidance of unpleasant or aversive activities is itself a reinforcer (negative) for behavior.

In effect, the parents acquiesce to the child and the child succeeds in failing to accomplish the requested activity. In some instances, the child leaves the situation; he may run out of the room or yard without performing the task. Or the parent may storm out of the room in anger or frustration, leaving the child to return to his previous activities. In some cases, the parents may in fact complete the command themselves, as when a parent picks up the toys for the child. Or the parent may assist the child with the task after directing the child to do so. In some instances, the child succeeds in not only escaping from doing the task but also in receiving a positive consequence as well. For example, when a parent directs a child to pick up toys, the child refuses, throws himself to the floor, and begins hitting his head against the floor. Out of fear that the child may injure himself, the parent may respond by picking the child up and holding him while trying to soothe him. As a result, the child's tantrum and self-injurious behavior are not only negatively reinforced by an escape from the unpleasant task initially requested by the parent but also positively reinforced by the attention from the parent. It is likely that such dual reinforcement for oppositional behavior rapidly accelerates children's acquisition and maintenance of such behavior patterns in future similar circumstances.

Parents' acquiescent interaction patterns can be found to underlie many of the negative encounters between parents and defiant children. They must be the focus of treatment if the complaints of the family are to be successfully ameliorated and the future risks of maladjustment to the children reduced.

Situational Pervasiveness

Defiance spreads, much like a cancer, from the home into other settings. Research suggests that children who display defiant behavior in one situation are highly likely to employ it eventually elsewhere, reacting to other commands or instructions and to other adults or children as they do to their parents. Failing to take steps to improve child defiance may therefore have effects across many situations and individuals.

Effects on Family Social Ecology

Defiant behavior by a child, as outlined in Figure 1, may have indirect effects on family functioning that may, reciprocally come back to have further detrimental effects on the psychological adjustment of the defiant child. From impaired management practices the parents use with a defiant child, the child acquires a set of coercive behaviors that he or she uses against the parents and other family members or even peers when instructed to do something he or she does not like to do. From those rare occasions where yelling, threatening, or punishing the child has eventually led to compliance by the child, parents may acquire a set of rapidly escalating coercive behaviors to use with the child. Furthermore, over time parents may come to issue progressively fewer commands, knowing in advance that the child will meet them with resistant, oppositional behavior. Parents instead may assume more of the child's chores and responsibilities or assign them to a more compliant sibling. This situation may then lead not only to a decline in the child's overall level of successful adaptive functioning (i.e., independence, self-care, degree of responsibleness, and so on) but to the development in siblings of hostility and resentment toward the defiant child because the defiant child has comparatively less work to do.

In some cases, parents and siblings spend progressively less leisure time and initiate fewer recreational pursuits with the defiant child so as to avoid unpleasant encounters. Siblings may acquire and use repertoires of coercive behavior toward the defiant child as well as toward parents; after all, parents frequently employ coercive tactics with other members of the family, not just the clinic-referred defiant child.

Thus, the density of aversive social events in the families of defiant children is often substantially higher than normal. The effects of such patterns in a family on one's self-esteem as a parent, on family harmony, on marital harmony, should the child oppose one parent more than the other, or on the self-esteem of the defiant child goes almost without saying. In the parent–child relations of defiant children, the behavior of parent and child affect each other reciprocally while also resulting in spillover effects on the social ecology of the whole family.

Developmental Persistence

Defiant behavior in children appears to be highly stable over time. In fact, it may be one of the most stable of childhood behavioral disorders across development.

Prediction of Diverse Negative Developmental Outcomes

Targeting early defiant behavior for treatment is important because of its repeated association in research with maladjustments during the adolescent and young adult years. Defiant and coercive behavior, especially if it is of such magnitude and duration that it leads to clinical referral, is a precursor of the development of other more serious forms of antisocial behavior, criminal activity, and substance abuse. Childhood oppositional behavior also significantly predicts later problems with academic performance and peer acceptance. The risk for later depression, suicidal ideation, and suicide attempts is also greater in children with defiant or aggressive behavior.

In fact, research is showing that the presence of oppositional defiant behavior in children is a more significant predictor of a widespread array of negative social and academic risks than are most other forms of deviant child behavior. The developmental risks become even more likely and more adverse when childhood defiant behavior is accompanied by higher levels of ADHD symptoms, particularly childhood impulsivity. Oppositional behavior, therefore, must be taken seriously and be treated.

Important Aspects of the Interactions of Defiant Children with Their Parents

The body of research on relations between defiant children and their parents is too great to review here, but because the more consistent and general findings from this research are important to consider in understanding and treating defiant children and their families, I summarize them here.

Without a doubt, research repeatedly demonstrates that the quality or nature of parent–child interactions is strongly and reliably associated with childhood noncompliant, defiant, and aggressive behavior patterns, the persistence of these behaviors over development, and the risk for later adolescent delinquency. The attachment relationships to their parents of children with oppositional behavior are of a poor quality. The parents of defiant children provide highly inconsistent and, at times, even positive consequences to children for their deviant behavior. Poor attachment, unpredictable consequences, and inadvertent reinforcement of defiant behavior may serve to increase and sustain occurrences of oppositional child behavior. When children act out, throw temper tantrums, or directly oppose commands, it is surely difficult not to attend to such behavior. But even though attention may seem negative to the parents, it may still serve to increase future oppositional behavior. Parents may provide positive attention or rewards to children in an effort to get them to stop "making a scene" in a store, restaurant, or other public place. Buying a child a candy bar for throwing a tantrum over initially not getting it is but one obvious way in which parents may accelerate the acquisition and maintenance of deviant child behavior.

Conversely, parents may also provide less attention and reinforcement for prosocial or appropriate behaviors of the child. Clinical experience suggests that parents of deviant children monitor or survey child behaviors less than parents of normal children, so they are not always aware of ongoing appropriate child behaviors. Even if they are aware that the child is behaving well, they may elect not to attend to the child or praise him for several reasons. One is that many parents report that when they praise or attend to good behavior in their child, it provokes a burst of negative behavior from the child. This leads the parents to "let sleeping dogs lie" when they encounter ongoing acceptable child behavior. It has neither been established that this burst of negative child behavior occurs when parents try to praise a behavior problem child nor, if it does, what the learning history was that established this behavioral pattern. It is possible that parental praise for good behavior in a child prompts the child to misbehave to continue the parental attention. Had the child continued to behave well, the parent might have terminated the interaction, moving on to do something else.

Another reason parents fail to react positively when a defiant child behaves well is that they dislike interacting with the child at all and avoid interacting with the child when possible. Parents of a chronically defiant child often develop animosity or "grudges" toward the child and so do not praise the child when the child finally behaves well. Eventually parents spend significantly less leisure and recreational time with the defiant child simply because it is not fun to do so.

Parents of oppositional children, especially children at risk for later delinquency, who monitor their children's activities infrequently also attend less to unacceptable behavior. As in the saying "out of sight, out of mind," parents may eventually reduce the amount of effort they spend monitoring a child's behavior so that they do not to have to confront unacceptable behavior. By overlooking problem behavior, they do not have to face the aversiveness of another negative, coercive exchange with the child. This may explain the frequent clinical observation that some parents seem to be oblivious to ongoing negative behavior occurring in their presence—behavior other parents would react to in a corrective fashion.

For whatever reason, some parents of oppositional children are simply not invested in serving as parents to their children, possibly because of their own younger than normal age when becoming parents, their social immaturity, their limited intelligence, or even their own psychological or psychiatric disorders. Regardless of its origins, a decline in parental monitoring and management of child conduct is associated with the development of some of the most serious forms of conduct disorder—both covert antisocial behavior, such as lying, stealing, and destruction of community property, and overt antisocial acts, such as physical aggression towards others.

Parents sometimes actually punish appropriate child behavior, possibly because of resentment that may have developed over years of negative interactions with the child. Parents give a child "back-handed" compliments for finally doing something correctly, as when they sarcastically remark, "It's about time you cleaned your room; why couldn't you do that yesterday?"

Inconsistent and unpredictable punishing of both prosocial and antisocial child behavior, as well as intermittent and unpredictable rewarding of both classes of child behavior, has been referred to as "indiscriminant" parenting: The children are damned if they do and damned if they don't comply. This form of indiscriminant use of consequences by parents creates a great deal of social unpredictability in families and especially in the parent–child relationship. Families experience such environments as inherently aversive. In such a situation, any response by the child that could be instrumental in reducing unpredictability is negatively reinforced and thereby increases in frequency. Thus, children come to use forms of defiant and aggressive behavior toward parents that increase predictability in the course of parent–child interactions.

Both parents and children in families with defiant children are negatively reinforced for behaving in aggressive and coercive ways toward each other. The negative behavior of one member of the parent–child dyad serves to terminate the ongoing negative behavior of the other thereby reinforcing the first member's coercive behavior. This may explain why parents and children, once having begun a negative interaction with each other, escalate their negative behavior toward each other very quickly to intense levels of aggression or coercion. Furthermore, the likelihood that such forms of interaction will occur again is greatly increased as a result.

It is necessary to remember that negative reinforcement is *not* the same as punishment. Negative reinforcement is said to occur when, during a situation where the child is subjected to aversive, unpleasant, or otherwise negative stimuli, the child displays a behavior that successfully terminates the aversive situation or permits him to escape from future such situations. For instance, a child often finds aversive the attempt of a parent to make the child get ready for bed while the child is watching a favorite television program. The child may oppose, resist, or otherwise escape the parental command through defiant, aggressive, or other coercive behavior that delays having to get ready for bed. The child's success at escaping the command, even if only temporary, negatively reinforces the oppositional behavior. The likelihood of the child resisting the command the next time the parent asks the child to get ready for bed has increased. The more a parent repeats the request, the more intense the child's resistance becomes due to previous success at escaping or avoiding the activity specified in the command. As already noted, parents eventually often acquiesce to this type of coercive behavior. Parents need not acquiesce every time for a child to acquire resistant behavior.

Parents may acquire aggressive or coercive behavior toward their defiant child by much the same process. A parent may have been successful on occasion at getting the child to cease whining, refusing, or throwing a tantrum and to comply with a command through the parent's use of yelling, screaming, or even physical aggression against the child. The parent may also have discovered that rapidly increasing the intensity of the negative behavior toward the child is more successful at getting the child to capitulate and obey if the child initially opposes the command. Hence, in subsequent situations the parent may escalate very quickly to intense negative behavior toward the child. Success with this strategy every time or even the majority of times is not necessary to reinforce this type of parental behavior across most command–compliance encounters with the defiant child; only occasional success with coercive behavior is needed to sustain this type of behavior.

Viewed from this perspective, both parent and child have a history of periodic but partial success at escaping or avoiding each other's escalating aversive or coercive behavior. As a result, each continues to employ it with the other in most command–compliance interactions. Over time, each learns that when a command–compliance situation arises, the faster each escalates negative emotional intensity and coerciveness, the more likely the other is to acquiesce to demands. As a result, confrontational interactions between parent and child may escalate quickly to intense, emotional, and even aggressive confrontations, which, on some occasions, may end with physical abuse of the child by the parent, destruction of property by the child, assault by the child on the parent, or even self-injury by the child.

Obviously, much defiant child behavior is not sustained by positive attention or reinforcement from the parent but by negative reinforcement or the desire to escape from unwanted, unpleasant, or aversive conditions the parent is attempting to impose on the child. Accordingly, when a parent ignores defiant child behavior, it may only worsen the problem, as the child is likely to view the parent's behavior as acquiescence. In many cases, parents cannot ignore the child because in so doing the child escapes from performing the parental command. Parents in such a situation have to continue interacting with the child if they wish to get the task accomplished. Many experienced clinicians have noted this problem in training parents of defiant children—ignoring defiant behavior is not always either successful or possible. How to give *mild and consistent* punishment must be incorporated into any parent training program, as must prevention of the child from escaping the parental command, if the training is to be successful in diminishing child defiance that has developed through negative reinforcement.

This review of several important aspects of the interactions of defiant children with their parents has a number of implications for the training of parents in effective child management procedures, discussed in the other videotape in this series, *Managing the Defiant Child*. Parents must be trained to:

1. Increase the value of their attention and its worth in motivating and reinforcing their child's positive behavior
2. Increase positive attention and incentives for compliance while decreasing inadvertent punishment they provide for occasional compliance
3. Decrease the amount of inadvertent positive attention they provide for negative behavior
4. Increase the use of immediate and consistent mild punishment for occurrences of noncompliance

5. Insure that escape from the activity required of the child does not occur (i.e., ensure that the child eventually complies with the command)
6. Reduce the frequency of repeat commands to avoid delays in compliance (act, don't yak)
7. Recognize and rapidly terminate escalating and confronting negative interactions with the child
8. Increase the monitoring of the child's behavior to ensure discipline of the violation of parental or societal rules and the reward of displays of compliance and appropriate social conduct

All of this, then, should serve to reduce the unpredictability involved in indiscriminant parenting while ensuring that child coercive behaviors are unsuccessful in escaping or avoiding parental requests, demands, and commands.

What Causes Defiance in Children?

As we've said, one of the major causes of noncompliance, defiance, and social aggression repeatedly identified in research studies is the poor, ineffective, inconsistent, and indiscriminate child management methods of parents, often combined with unusually harsh but inconsistent disciplinary methods and poor monitoring of child activities. As a result, defiance by children becomes a very effective method for escaping or avoiding unpleasant, boring, or effortful tasks, perhaps increasing the predictability of consequences in parent–child exchanges (no matter how negative), and on some occasions even obtaining rewards (e.g., candy for the tantrum in the store). But it would be erroneous to conclude that all defiant behavior results from the parent–child relationship. While the exact form of the defiant behavior and even its severity probably has much to do with the child's learning history in a family, the probability of acquiring or displaying oppositional behavior is also affected by at least three other domains of influence. Impaired child and family management practices, and the three other causal influences make up a *four-factor model* of oppositional behavior in children.

Impaired Child and Family Management Practices

This is the inconsistent, indiscriminate, and often hostile approach to child management discussed in the previous section. Often accompanied by reduced overall behavior monitoring both inside and outside the home, poor child management skills can easily train a child to become defiant.

Temperament of the Child

It is becoming clear that children of certain temperaments and cognitive characteristics are more prone to display coercive and aggressive behavior and to be noncompliant than are other children. In particular, children who are prone to emotional responses (high emotionality), are often irritable, have poor habit regulation, are highly active, and/or are more inattentive and impulsive seem to be more likely to display disruptive behavior disorders and, therefore, to demonstrate defiant and coercive behavior than are children who do not have such negative characteristics of temperament. While parental psychopathology and poor marital and family functioning may further exacerbate a child's risks for greater defiance and aggression, negative temperamental features are among the strongest influences in this process and may be sufficient in themselves to create the risks. The effects of early childhood temperament may be gender-specific: Negative temperament in infant and toddler boys may predict higher risk for later oppositional behavior, whereas, for toddler girls, early negative temperament may predict a *decrease* in the risk for later aggressive behavior but possibly an increase in later risk for internalizing disorders, such as anxiety or depression.

Symptoms of ADHD, such as overactivity, inattention, and impulsivity, are typically considered aspects of temperament in infants and toddlers. Should they persist into preschool years and eventually school age, such symptoms are likely to create parent–child interaction conflicts. Symptoms of ADHD may prevent a child from finishing assigned activities and thus are likely to elicit increased commands, supervision, and negative reactions from parents. Children with higher levels of ADHD symptoms may also be likely to respond to reprimands and parental confrontations with negative emotional reactions. The co-occurrence of ADHD symptoms, particularly poor impulse control, with early oppositional behavior is especially virulent, predicting significantly greater family conflicts and worse developmental outcomes, particularly in the realm of later antisocial activity, than does either dimension of behavior alone.

Temperament of the Parents

The probability of defiance in children may increase as a result of similar temperamental and cognitive characteristics in the child's parents. Immature, inexperienced, impulsive, inattentive, depressed, hostile, rejecting, or otherwise negatively temperamental parents are more likely to have defiant and aggressive children. This may be because they display inconsistent management strategies, show irritability and hostility toward their children, and provide little reinforcement for prosocial behavior. Through inconsistent and indiscriminate parenting, children experience periodic success at avoiding demands, further reinforcing oppositional or coercive behavior. Such increases in child coercive behavior may then feed back to further detrimentally affect parent mood, sense of competence, self-esteem, and even marital functioning in a vicious, reciprocal circle of effects. Such parents may also employ coercive behavior with others in the family, providing a model of negative behavior for the child to imitate. In particular, the level of maternal depression and maternal and paternal psychopathology, especially antisocial personality disorder or criminality, are significantly associated with risk for childhood oppositional and aggressive behavior and later delinquency.

Setting and Stress Events

It is also possible that larger contextual events surrounding the family, both internal and external, create or contribute to increased risks for child defiant behavior and aggression as well as later delinquency. As noted earlier, maternal social isolation is one such factor, as is maternal marital status. Single mothers are the most likely to have significantly aggressive children, followed in likelihood by mothers living with male partners but who are unmarried, and married mothers. These associations are moderated somewhat by higher social class. Marital discord also has been repeatedly linked to child disruptive and defiant behavior, although debate continues over the mechanisms involved in this relationship. Also, as noted earlier, family social disadvantage or social adversity is associated with risks for childhood defiant and aggressive behavior. All these aspects of the family setting contribute to parental inconsistency, indiscriminacy, and irritability in child management methods, which predisposes children to develop or sustain noncompliance or defiance in family interactions.

Many families referred for treatment of a defiant child have most or all of these predisposing characteristics: temperamental, impulsive, active, and inattentive children being raised by immature, temperamental, and impulsive parents in a family setting of marital, financial, health, or personal distress, where management of the child is characterized by inconsistent, harsh, indiscriminate, and coercive parenting often accompanied by reduced parental monitoring of the child's activities.

Summary

This manual describes the importance of defiance in children and the reasons it requires parental and professional concern and treatment. The processes whereby children develop, maintain, or increase their rate of oppositional, defiant, or noncompliant behavior are discussed in some detail. It appears that such behavior is chiefly sustained by its success in terminating parental demands and allowing the child to escape or avoid generally unpleasant, effortful, or boring tasks assigned by parents while often permitting the child to continue in a previous more desirable activity. Parents may escalate their rates of negative behavior toward the child because of the behavior's occasional success in terminating ongoing unpleasant child behavior and getting eventual child compliance. Both parents and children may be predisposed toward coercive behavior because of their temperamental patterns and psychological disorders. Family settings that include stress, marital discord, or parental social isolation, may serve to increase the probability of defiant child behavior because of the negative effect these events have on the consistency of parental management of the child, the positive reinforcement of compliant child behavior, and the general monitoring of child activities by parents.

Understanding the Defiant Child   21

APPENDIX

The following forms represent part of a packet of questionnaires sent to parents and teachers following their call to a clinic but prior to their scheduled appointment. This assessment process is described in more detail and available in reproducible form in my book *Defiant Children* (2nd ed.): *A Clinician's Manual for Assessment and Parent Training* (Barkley, 1997b, 1997c).

Developmental and Medical History

PREGNANCY AND DELIVERY

A. Length of pregnancy (e.g., full term, 40 weeks, 32 weeks, etc.) _____
B. Length of delivery (number of hours from initial labor pains to birth) _____
C. Mother's age when child was born _____
D. Child's birth weight _____
E. Did any of the following conditions occur during pregnancy/delivery?
   1. Bleeding — No Yes
   2. Excessive weight gain (more than 30 lbs.) — No Yes
   3. Toxemia/preeclampsia — No Yes
   4. Rh factor incompatibility — No Yes
   5. Frequent nausea or vomiting — No Yes
   6. Serious illness or injury — No Yes
   7. Took prescription medications — No Yes
      a. If Yes, name of medication _____
   8. Took illegal drugs — No Yes
   9. Used alcoholic beverage — No Yes
      a. If Yes, approximate number of drinks per week _____
   10. Smoked cigarettes — No Yes
       a. If Yes, approximate number of cigarettes per day (e.g., ½ pack) _____
   11. Was given medication to ease labor pains? — No Yes
       a. If Yes, name of medication _____
   12. Delivery was induced — No Yes
   13. Forceps were used during delivery — No Yes
   14. Had a breech delivery — No Yes
   15. Had a cesarean section delivery — No Yes

(cont.)

16. Other problems—please describe   No   Yes

F. Did any of the following conditions affect your child during delivery or within the first few days after birth?
1. Injured during delivery   No   Yes
2. Cardiopulmonary distress during delivery   No   Yes
3. Delivered with cord around neck   No   Yes
4. Had trouble breathing following delivery   No   Yes
5. Needed oxygen   No   Yes
6. Was cyanotic, turned blue   No   Yes
7. Was jaundiced, turned yellow   No   Yes
8. Had an infection   No   Yes
9. Had seizures   No   Yes
10. Was given medications   No   Yes
11. Born with a congenital defect   No   Yes
12. Was in hospital more than 7 days   No   Yes

INFANT HEALTH AND TEMPERAMENT

A. During the first 12 months, was your child:
1. Difficult to feed   No   Yes
2. Difficult to get to sleep   No   Yes
3. Colicky   No   Yes
4. Difficult to put on a schedule   No   Yes
5. Alert   No   Yes
6. Cheerful   No   Yes
7. Affectionate   No   Yes
8. Sociable   No   Yes
9. Easy to comfort   No   Yes
10. Difficult to keep busy   No   Yes
11. Overactive, in constant motion   No   Yes
12. Very stubborn, challenging   No   Yes

EARLY DEVELOPMENTAL MILESTONES

A. At what age did your child first accomplish the following:
1. Sitting without help   _____
2. Crawling   _____
3. Walking alone, without assistance   _____
4. Using single words (e.g., "mama," "dada," "ball," etc.)   _____
5. Putting two or more words together (e.g., "mama up")   _____
6. Bowel training, day and night   _____
7. Bladder training, day and night   _____

HEALTH HISTORY
A. Date of child's last physical exam: _____
B. At any time has your child had the following:

1. Asthma	Never	Past	Present
2. Allergies	Never	Past	Present
3. Diabetes, arthritis, or other chronic illnesses	Never	Past	Present
4. Epilepsy or seizure disorder	Never	Past	Present
5. Febrile seizures	Never	Past	Present
6. Chicken pox or other common childhood illnesses	Never	Past	Present
7. Heart or blood pressure problems	Never	Past	Present
8. High fevers (over 103°)	Never	Past	Present
9. Broken bones	Never	Past	Present
10. Severe cuts requiring stitches	Never	Past	Present
11. Head injury with loss of consciousness	Never	Past	Present
12. Lead poisoning	Never	Past	Present
13. Surgery	Never	Past	Present
14. Lengthy hospitalization	Never	Past	Present
15. Speech or language problems	Never	Past	Present
16. Chronic ear infections	Never	Past	Present
17. Hearing difficulties	Never	Past	Present
18. Eye or vision problems	Never	Past	Present
19. Fine motor/handwriting problems	Never	Past	Present
20. Gross motor difficulties, clumsiness	Never	Past	Present
21. Appetite problems (overeating or undereating)	Never	Past	Present
22. Sleep problems (falling asleep, staying asleep)	Never	Past	Present
23. Soiling problems	Never	Past	Present
24. Wetting problems	Never	Past	Present
25. Other health difficulties—please describe	Never	Past	Present

Disruptive Behavior Disorders Rating Scale—Parent Form

Child's name _____ Age _____ Date _____
Form completed by: _____
Relationship to child: (Circle one)
Mother   Father   Stepparent   Other: _____ (explain)

Instructions: Circle the number that *best describes* your child's behavior at home over the past 6 months.

	Never or rarely	Sometimes	Often	Very often
1. Fails to give close attention to details or makes careless mistakes in schoolwork	0	1	2	3
2. Has difficulty sustaining attention in tasks or play activities	0	1	2	3
3. Does not seem to listen when spoken to directly	0	1	2	3
4. Does not follow through on instructions and fails to finish work	0	1	2	3
5. Has difficulty organizing tasks and activities	0	1	2	3
6. Avoids tasks (e.g., schoolwork, homework) that require mental effort	0	1	2	3
7. Loses things necessary for tasks or activities	0	1	2	3
8. Is easily distracted	0	1	2	3
9. Is forgetful in daily activities	0	1	2	3
10. Fidgets with hands or feet or squirms in seat	0	1	2	3
11. Leaves seat in classroom or in other situations in which remaining seated is expected	0	1	2	3
12. Runs about or climbs excessively in situations in which it is inappropriate	0	1	2	3
13. Has difficulty playing or engaging in leisure activities quietly	0	1	2	3

14. Is "on the go" or acts as if "driven by a motor"	0	1	2	3
15. Talks excessively	0	1	2	3
16. Blurts out answers before questions have been completed	0	1	2	3
17. Has difficulty awaiting turn	0	1	2	3
18. Interrupts or intrudes on others	0	1	2	3
19. Loses temper	0	1	2	3
20. Argues with adults	0	1	2	3
21. Actively defies or refuses to comply with adults' requests or rules	0	1	2	3
22. Deliberately annoys people	0	1	2	3
23. Blames others for his/her mistakes or misbehavior	0	1	2	3
24. Is touchy or easily annoyed by others	0	1	2	3
25. Is angry and resentful	0	1	2	3
26. Is spiteful or vindictive	0	1	2	3

Instructions: Please indicate whether your child has done any of these activities in the past 12 months.

1. Often bullied, threatened, or intimidated others	No	Yes
2. Often initiated physical fights	No	Yes
3. Used a weapon that can cause serious physical harm to others (e.g., a bat, brick, broken bottle, knife, or gun)	No	Yes
4. Has been physically cruel to people	No	Yes
5. Has been physically cruel to animals	No	Yes
6. Has stolen while confronting a victim (e.g., mugging, purse snatching, extortion, armed robbery)	No	Yes
7. Has forced someone into sexual activity	No	Yes
8. Has deliberately engaged in fire setting with the intention of causing serious damage	No	Yes
9. Has deliberately destroyed others' property (other than by fire setting)	No	Yes
10. Has broken into someone else's house, building, or car	No	Yes
11. Often lies to obtain goods or favors or to avoid obligations (i.e., "cons" others)	No	Yes

(cont.)

12. Has stolen items of nontrivial value without confronting a victim (e.g., shoplifting, but without breaking and entering; forgery)   No   Yes

13. Often stays out at night despite parental prohibitions   No   Yes
If so, at what age did this begin? _____

14. Has run away from home overnight at least twice while living in parent's home, foster care, or group home   No   Yes
If so, how many times? _____

15. Is often truant from school   No   Yes
If so, at what age did he/she begin doing this? _____

Suggested Readings

American Psychiatric Association (1994). *Diagnostic and statistical manual of mental disorders* (4th ed.). Washington, DC: Author.
Barkley, R. A. (1990). *Attention deficit hyperactivity disorder: A handbook for diagnosis and treatment.* New York: Guilford Press.
Barkley, R. A. (1993a). *ADHD—What do we know?* [Video]. New York: Guilford Press.
Barkley, R. A. (1993b). *ADHD—What can we do?* [Video]. New York: Guilford Press.
Barkley, R. A. (1994a). *ADHD in the classroom* [Video]. New York: Guilford Press.
Barkley, R. A. (1994b). *ADHD in adults* [Video]. New York: Guilford Press.
Barkley, R. A. (1995). *Taking charge of ADHD: The complete authoritative guide for parents.* New York: Guilford Press.
Barkley, R. A. (1997a). *Managing the defiant child* [video]. New York: Guilford Press.
Barkley, R. A. (1997b). *Defiant children: A clinician's manual for assessment and parent training* (2nd ed.). New York: Guilford Press.
Barkley, R. A. (1997c). *Niño desafiantes: Materiales de evaluación y folletos para los padres* [Evaluation materials and handouts for parents from *Defiant children* (2nd ed.): *A clinician's manual for assessment and parent training*] (J. Bauermeister, C. C. Salas-Serrano, M. Matos, G. Reina, & D. Avila-Lopez, Trans.). New York: Guilford Press.
Dangel, R. F., & Polster, R. A. (1984). *Parent training.* New York: Guilford Press.
Forehand, R., & McMahon, R. (1981). *Helping the noncompliant child: A clinician's guide to parent training.* New York: Guilford Press.
Forgatch, M., & Patterson, G. R. (1990). *Parents and adolescents living together.* Eugene, OR: Castalia.
Mash, E. J., & Barkley, R. A. (Eds.) (1996). *Child psychopathology.* New York: Guilford Press.
Mash, E. J., & Barkley, R. A. (Eds.) (1997). *Treatment of childhood disorders* (2nd ed.). New York: Guilford Press.
Patterson, G. R. (1982). *Coercive family process.* Eugene, OR: Castalia.
Patterson, G. R., Reid, J. B., & Dishion, T. J. (1992). *Antisocial boys.* Eugene, OR: Castalia.
Patterson, G. R., Reid, J. B., Jones, R. R., & Conger, R. E. (1975). *A social learning approach to family intervention* (Vol. 1). Eugene, OR: Castalia.
Robin, A. R., & Foster, S. (1989). *Negotiating parent-adolescent conflict.* New York: Guilford Press.

Webster-Stratton, C. & Spitzer, A. (1996). Parenting a young child with conduct problems. In T. H. Ollendick & R. J. Prinz (Eds.), *Advances in clinical child psychology* (Vol. 18, pp. 1–62). New York: Plenum.

Parent Training

The following national organizations may be contacted for referrals to local sources of information regarding parent training groups for oppositional defiance disorder.

The ADD Resource Center
215 West 75th Street
New York, NY 10023-1799
(212)721-0049

American Psychological Association
750 First Street NE
Washington, DC 20002
(800)374-2721

ChADD
499 NW 70th Avenue
Suite 109
Plantation, FL 33317
(305)587-3700

Council for Exceptional Children
1920 Association Drive
Reston, VA 20191
(703)620-3660

Learning Disabilities Association of America
4156 Library Road
Pittsburgh, PA 15234-1349
(412)341-1515

National Center for Learning Disabilities
381 Park Avenue South, Suite 401
New York, NY 10016
(212)545-7510

National Information Center for Children and Youth with Disabilities (NICHY)
P.O. Box 1492
Washington, DC 20013-1492
(800)695-0285